Narjes ABID
Soumaya BOUJNAH

E-cigarette use among medical students

Narjes ABID
Soumaya BOUJNAH

E-cigarette use among medical students

ScienciaScripts

Imprint

Any brand names and product names mentioned in this book are subject to trademark, brand or patent protection and are trademarks or registered trademarks of their respective holders. The use of brand names, product names, common names, trade names, product descriptions etc. even without a particular marking in this work is in no way to be construed to mean that such names may be regarded as unrestricted in respect of trademark and brand protection legislation and could thus be used by anyone.

Cover image: www.ingimage.com

This book is a translation from the original published under ISBN 978-620-6-72356-1.

Publisher:
Sciencia Scripts
is a trademark of
Dodo Books Indian Ocean Ltd. and OmniScriptum S.R.L publishing group

120 High Road, East Finchley, London, N2 9ED, United Kingdom
Str. Armeneasca 28/1, office 1, Chisinau MD-2012, Republic of Moldova, Europe
Printed at: see last page
ISBN: 978-620-8-13984-1

THANK YOU

To our Master and President of the Jury Professor Gargouri Imen

We are honoured that you have agreed to chair this jury and judge our dissertation.

We have always admired your knowledge, your skills, your kindness and your teaching qualities.

We would like to take this opportunity to express our deep gratitude, admiration and respect.

To our Master and Judge Professor Dr LOUKIL Manel

Thank you very much for the honour you have bestowed on us by agreeing to judge this work.

We have the utmost admiration for your great professional and human qualities.

May this work bear witness to our most respectful sentiments.

__To my dear friend and Judge Dr OMRANE Asma__

We are particularly touched by the honour you have done us by

agreeing to sit on the jury for this dissertation.

Working with you is both an honour and a pleasure.

Yours faithfully

To my Master and Supervisor Dr ABID Narjes

Thank you for entrusting us with this project.

You supervised us with a great deal of patience, rigour and availability.

We were particularly touched by your expertise and modesty.

We can't thank you enough for everything you've done to help us prepare this work.

TABLE OF CONTENTS

INTRODUCTION

Smoking is a major public health problem. It is one of the leading causes of preventable disease and premature death in the world (1). It is responsible for a number of serious diseases with high morbidity and mortality, and has a major impact on public health in terms of costs and absenteeism. According to the World Health Organisation (WHO) report published in 2023, tobacco consumption is responsible for more than 8 million deaths a year (2).

Tobacco control and prevention are major public health concerns. To combat this scourge, a range of medicinal and non-medicinal smoking cessation aids are currently available.

The electronic cigarette (e-cigarette), which uses a heating element vapourisation technique, was invented and patented in 2009. Since then, its use has grown exponentially around the world. It is often seen by the general public as an aid to smoking cessation. However, this remains a controversial issue, and learned societies have not yet included it in the therapeutic arsenal against nicotine addiction. In addition, a number of fears have arisen around it, given that its long-term harmful effects are not well understood, and that it could be associated with the initiation of smoking among adolescents and young adults.This is the background to our work, the aim of which was to study the practices and experiences of e-cigarette users among medical students, to analyse their expectations of this electronic device and to assess its influence on their smoking habits.

POPULATION AND METHOD

I. Type of study

This is a cross-sectional descriptive study.

II. Study population

1. Inclusion criteria

Medical students meeting these three criteria were included

- Externs, interns, residents or thesis candidates belonging to one of

the four faculties of medicine in the Republic of Tunisia

- Smoking or having smoked electronic cigarettes

- And who completed the study's self-questionnaire.

2. Non-inclusion criteria

Medical students who only smoke conventional tobacco and have

never smoked an electronic cigarette.

III. Methods

1. Conduct of the survey

The survey was conducted using a self-administered questionnaire

developed on Google Forms and distributed online via social networks

(Facebook) and accessible via the following link

https://docs.google.com/forms/d/e/1FAIpQLSfzNcbqbK1NafGU7k_Eu

uolg41GEZz4cBGUkY

rUck_ZVrO7ew/viewform?fbclid=IwAR3ZeDMKfukDoj5p2ixZcoFK

6UZY205XPzMd6wg81 v66vsjZAS21LvOEzI

2. Data collection

The self-questionnaire sent to medical students included a preamble

explaining the purpose of the study. It also contained three parts, as

detailed below.

• Socio-demographic and professional data

The following were collected:

- Age

- The genre

- The original medical school

- Speciality and level of study

• Characteristics of smoking habits

The following data were collected:

- Classic smokers (age of onset, intensity, duration)

- Consumption of other psychoactive substances

- Characteristics of e-cigarette use (age of first vaping, frequency of
vaping, switch from vaping to conventional tobacco, reason for
vaping, concentration and flavour of e-liquid used, etc.).

• **The beliefs and expectations of the population studied
regarding electronic cigarettes**

- The influence of vaping on normal tobacco consumption (cessation
or reduction in consumption)

- Undesirable effects experienced as a result of using electronic
cigarettes

- The beliefs of the population studied about the use of e-cigarettes

a. **Statistical analysis**

Data were collected using Excel and retransmitted using SPSS version
22. The descriptive and analytical study was carried out using SPSS
software. The significance level was set at 0.05.

b. **Bibliographic research**

The bibliographic search was carried out using PubMed, Science
Direct and the Google Scholar search engine.

The keywords used were: smoking, electronic cigarettes, medical
students, smoking cessation.

RESULTS

I. DESCRIPTIVE STUDY

Our study involved 31 medical students who use or have used electronic cigarettes.

1. Socio-demographic characteristics of the study population

a. Breakdown by age

The mean age of our study population was 28±4 years, with extremes ranging from 22 to 45 years.

b. Breakdown by gender

Our sample comprised 23 men (74.2%) and 8 women (25.8%). The gender ratio was 2.87 (Figure 1).

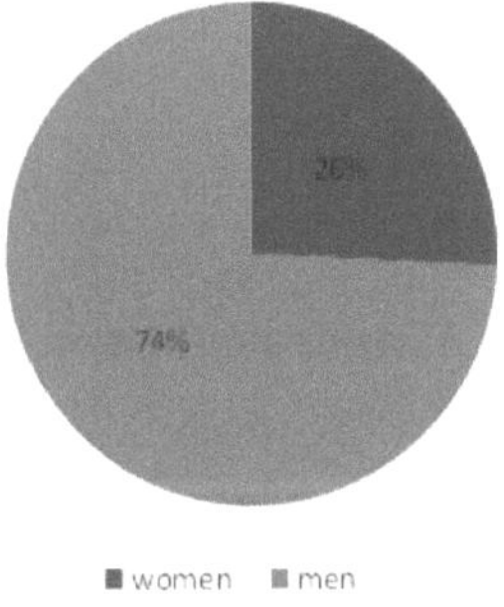

Figure 1: Breakdown of the study population by gender

c. Breakdown by faculty of origin

The majority of study participants (54.8%) were from the Tunisian Faculty of Medicine (Figure 2).

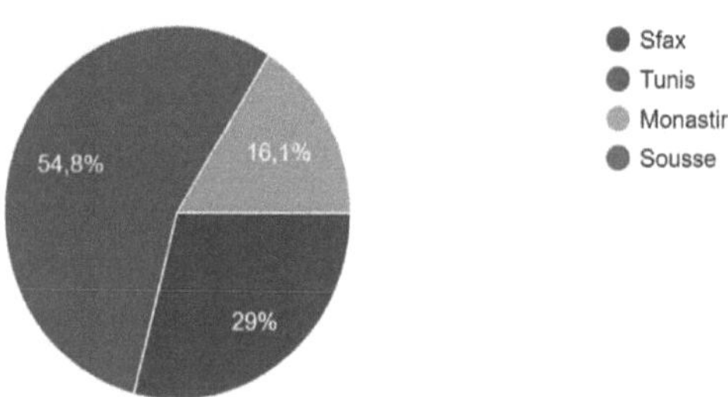

Figure 2: Breakdown of study population by faculty of origin

d. Breakdown by level of education

Of the participants, 77.4% were medical residents (Figure 3).

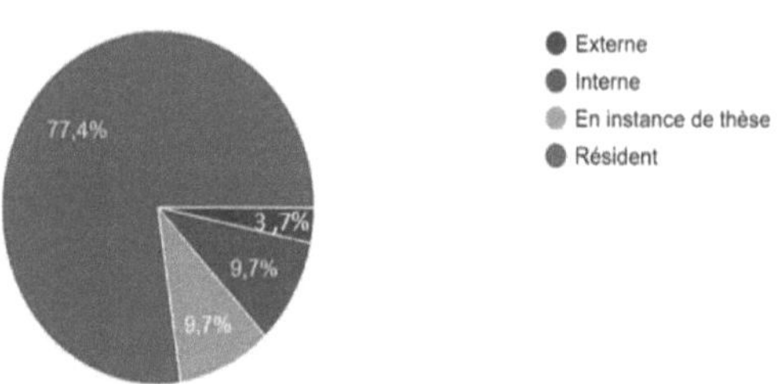

Figure 3: Breakdown of study population by level of education

2. Characteristics of the smoking habits of the population studied

a. Smoking tobacco

Twenty-three participants were smokers (74.2%). Seven of these participants had already stopped smoking before they started vaping (Figure 4).

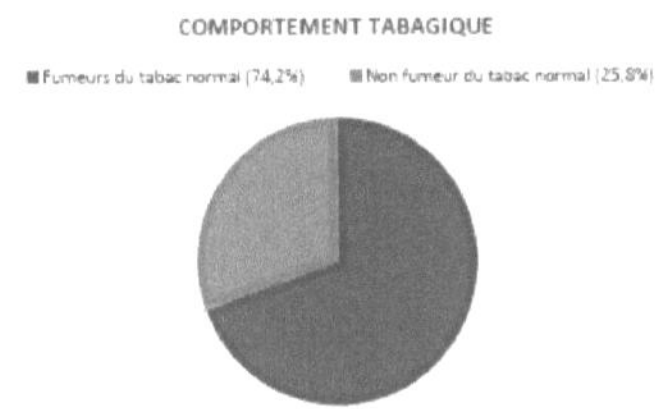

**Figure 4: Breakdown of the population studied according to
smoking habits**

The average age of onset of smoking was 21±4 years, with extremes ranging from 15 to 28 years.In almost half the cases (n=16; 51.6%) smoking had begun before the age of 20 years old. The average duration of smoking was 7.59 years at the time of the survey, with extremes ranging from 3 to 20 years. Almost a fifth (19.4%) of regular smokers smoked more than 20 cigarettes a day (Figure 5).

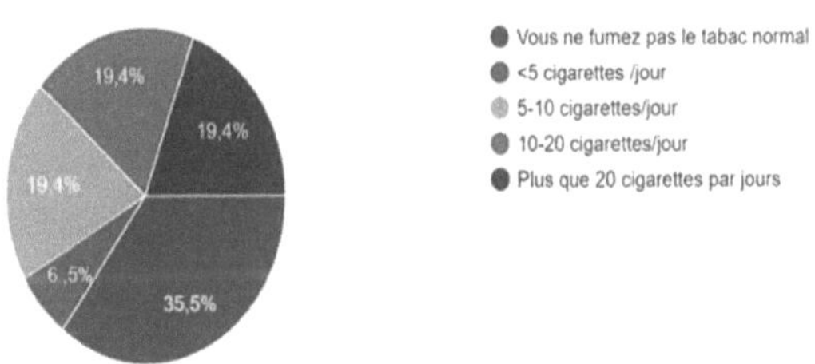

**Figure 5: Breakdown of the population studied according to the
number of cigarettes smoked per day**

b. Consumption of other psychoactive substances

E-cigarette use was associated with the use of other psychoactive substances in 16.1% of cases (5 participants) (Figure 6): alcohol in 2 cases, cannabis in 2 cases and a psychoactive drug (3,4-methylenedioxy-N-methylamphetamine, commonly known as Ectasy) in 1 case.

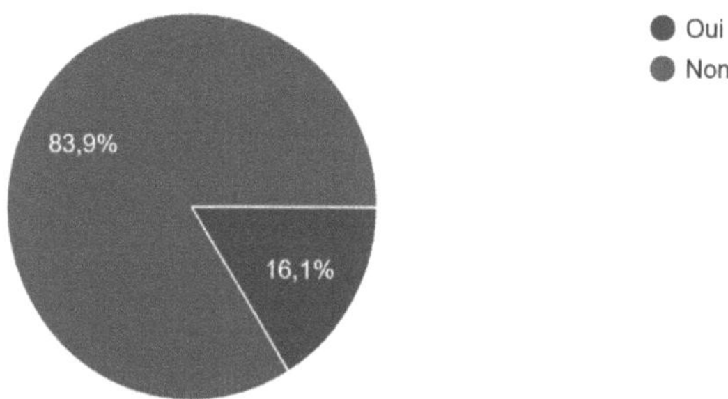

Figure 6: Breakdown of the population studied by consumption of psychoactive substances other than tobacco smoked

c. Characteristics of electronic cigarette consumption

i. Age of first vapour

The average age of first use of electronic cigarettes was 26.25±4.9 years [17-43 years]. Fifteen participants (48.3%) had experimented with electronic cigarettes before the age of 25. Fifteen participants (48.4%) were not smokers of normal tobacco when they started vaping and sixteen smoked both electronic cigarettes and normal tobacco (51.6%).

ii. Frequency of electronic cigarette use

Twenty-one participants (37.7%) used electronic cigarettes on a daily basis, with 64.5% using them several times a day. A third of the participants (32.3%) used it only a few times a week (Figure 7).

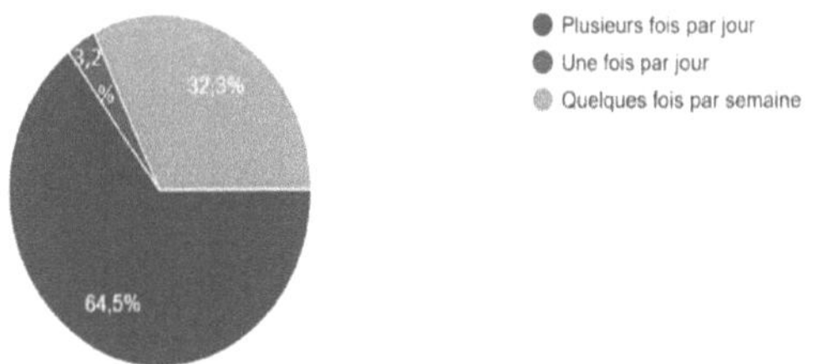

Figure 7: Breakdown of the study population by frequency of use of electronic cigarettes

Almost half of the participants (51.6%, n=16) increased their smoking frequency over time Around two-thirds of the subjects included in the study (20 participants; 64.5%) intend to stop using electronic cigarettes. A further eleven (35.5%) stopped using electronic cigarettes but resumed at a later date.

iii. Characteristics of the electronic cigarette

The concentration of nicotine in the e-liquid was 6 mg in 48.4% of cases. Almost a third of the participants (38.7%) stated that they did not know the concentration of nicotine in their e-cigarette. Three students used electronic cigarettes containing no nicotine (Figure 8).

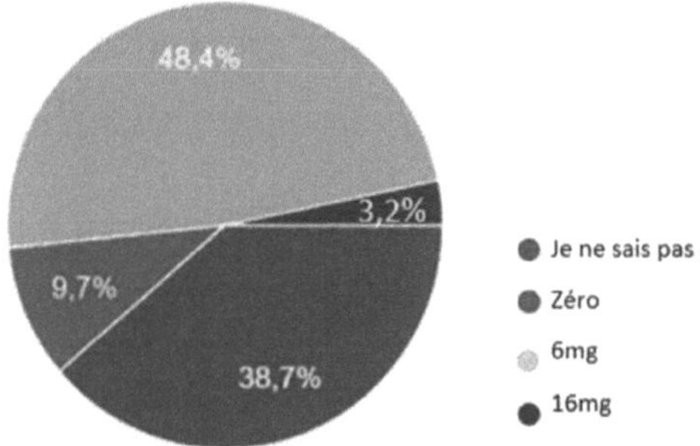

Figure 8: Breakdown of the population studied according to the nicotine concentration of the e-liquid

Fruit was the most commonly used flavour (58.1%), followed by mint (16.1%). Three participants used tobacco flavour (Figure 9).

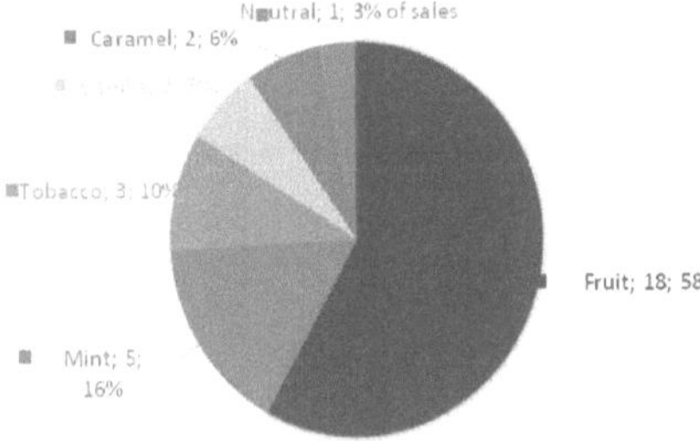

Figure 9: Breakdown of the population studied according to the flavour used for the electronic cigarette

iv. Reasons for using electronic cigarettes

Among the 16 traditional tobacco smokers, twelve participants (39%) started vaping with a view to giving up smoking and four were looking for a better taste than tobacco. The reasons that led the others to start vaping were curiosity (11 participants (35.4%) and the influence of peers (4 participants,12.9%) (Figure 10).

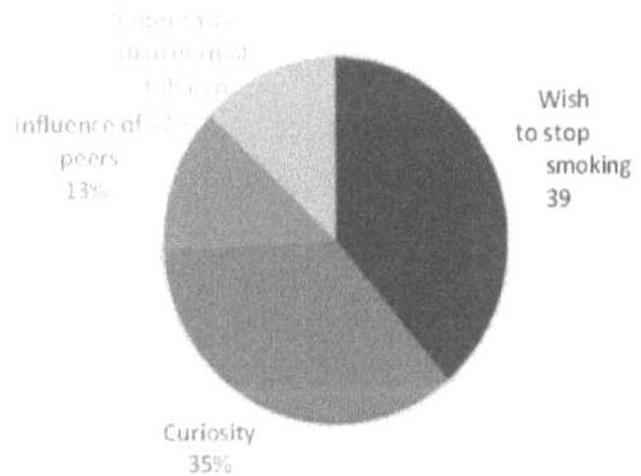

Figure 10: Breakdown of the population studied according to the reasons for using electronic cigarettes

3. E-cigarette beliefs and expectations of the population studied

a. Influence of vaping on tobacco consumption

i. Normal tobacco smokers

At the time of initiation of vaping, 16 participants were normal cigarette smokers (51.6%). Nine of them succeeded in reducing their tobacco consumption after using the e-cigarette and 3 participants succeeded in giving up smoking completely (Figure 11).

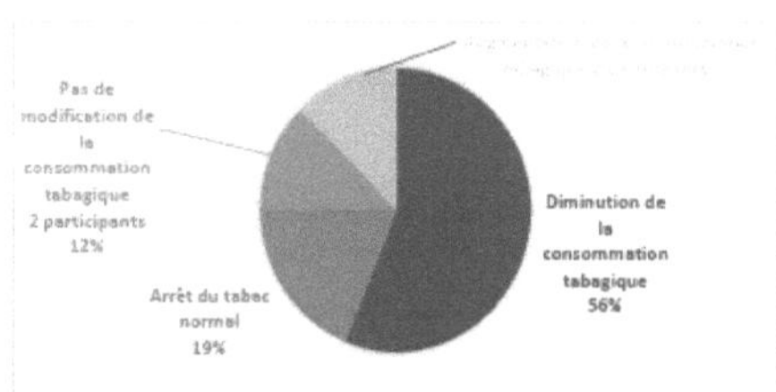

Figure 11: Influence of vaping on tobacco consumption among active smokers

ii. In non-smokers of normal tobacco :

Fifteen people were not smokers of normal tobacco when they first experimented with the electronic cigarette. Three of them wanted to switch to normal tobacco after they started vaping and 4 of them did switch to smoked tobacco.

b. Adverse reactions to electronic cigarettes

i. Psychological

Vaping made 67.7% of participants feel worried. The reasons for this feeling are detailed in table 1.

TABLE 1: Reasons for feeling worried about using electronic cigarettes

Cause for concern caused by smoking	N	%
Fears of harmful consequences of vapoatge on their health	11	35,5
Material expenses required for vaping	5	16,1
Feelings of guilt towards parents	5	16,1
Total	21	100

Almost half of the participants (45.2%) felt addicted to e-cigarettes (Figure 16).

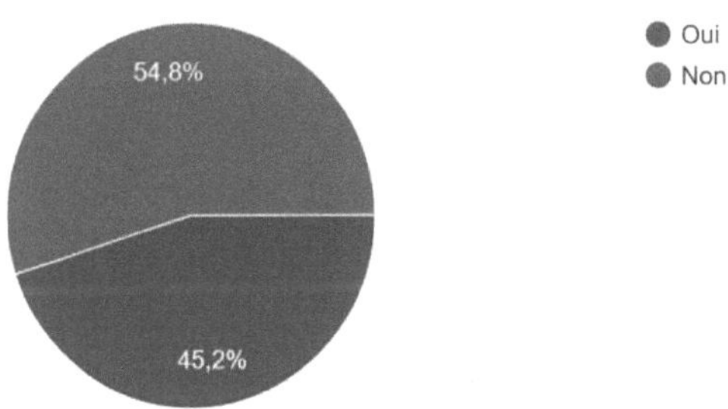

Figure 12: Feeling of dependence on electronic cigarettes

ii. Somatic (Table 2)

The majority of participants reported no adverse somatic effects secondary to e-cigarette use (19 cases, 61.2%). In the other cases (n=12, 38.7%), the main complaint was the dry cough present in 6 participants.

TABLE 2: Adverse reactions reported by e-cigarette users

Undesirable effects	N	%
Cough	6	50
Sore throats	1	8,3
Extinction of the voice	2	16,6
Headaches	1	8,3
Sneezing	1	8,3
Nausea and vomiting	1	8,3
Total	12	100%

c. Beliefs of the population studied on the use of e-cigarettes

According to our study, the majority of participants (74.2%) thought that e-cigarettes were less harmful than smoked tobacco, while 19.4% thought that e-cigarettes were as harmful as normal cigarettes (Figure 17).

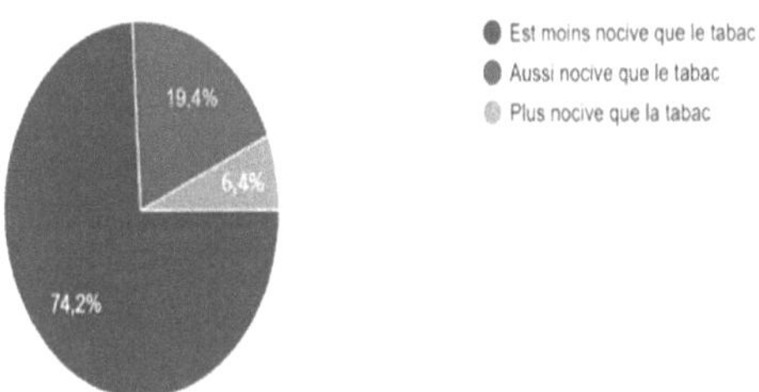

Figure 13: Beliefs of the population studied about the harmfulness of electronic cigarettes

Around two thirds of subjects (64.5%) thought that the electronic cigarette is a substitute for normal tobacco, and almost a third thought that the e-cigarette is more of a smoking cessation aid (Figure 18).

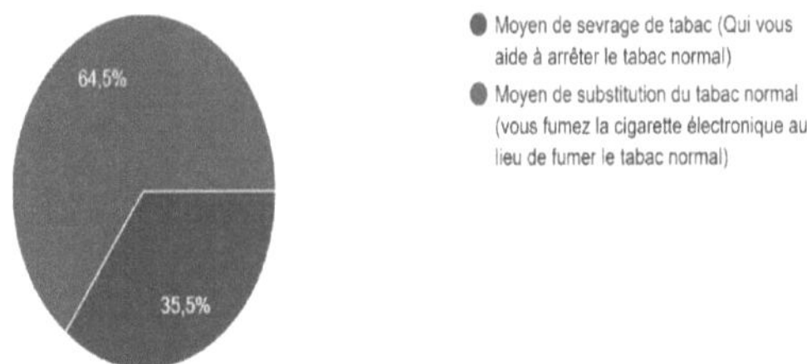

Figure 14: Beliefs about using electronic cigarettes

II. ANALYTICAL STUDY

1- Factors associated with daily use of electronic cigarettes

After analysing the data from our study, we find that the number of cigarettes smoked per day is correlated with daily consumption of e-cigarettes (p=0.044). In fact, a high number of cigarettes smoked per day is associated with daily consumption of e-cigarettes. No correlation was identified between daily e-cigarette use and gender, use of other substances, nicotine concentration or the beliefs of the subjects included in the study about the usefulness of vape (p>0.05) (Table 3).

Table 3: Factors associated with daily use of electronic cigarettes

Factor studied	p
Number of cigarettes smoked per day (>20 cig/d)	0,044
Sex (male)	0,660
Use of other substances psychoactive	0,0,64
Nicotine concentration	0,155
Beliefs about the use of electronic cigarettes as a means of withdrawal, substitution)	0,217

2- Factors associated with switching from vaping to normal cigarettes

The univariate analysis concluded that gender was a factor associated with switching from e-cigarettes to smoked tobacco (p=0.026). Male subjects were at greater risk of switching to regular cigarettes. However, the use of other psychoactive substances, multiday vape use, nicotine concentration and dependence were not associated with switching to smoked cigarettes, with p values of 0.467, 0.970, 0.236

and 0.871 respectively.

3-   Factors associated with feelings of anxiety about vaping

The analytical study analysed several factors with a view to finding a relationship between them and the anxiety felt by vapers. We found that the use of other psychoactive substances was associated with the feeling of guilt expressed by the respondents (p=0.028). Daily consumption of the e-cigarette, its nicotine concentration, the increase in consumption over time and the adverse effects reported were not associated with the feeling of anxiety reported (p>0.05) (Table 4).

Table 4: Factors associated with feelings of anxiety about vaping

Factor studied	P
Use of other substances psychoactive	0,028
Daily use of e-cigarettes	0,780
The concentration of nicotine in e-cigarettes	0,947
The increase in consumption of e-cigarettes over time	0,133
Reported adverse reactions	0,729

4- Factors influencing the desire to stop vaping

Univariate analysis identified that belief in the use of e-cigarettes was the factor influencing the desire to stop vaping (p=0.002). No statically significant relationship was found between the desire to stop using electronic cigarettes and the following parameters: age of onset of use (>20 years), frequency of vaping, consequences on psychological state (feelings of guilt/dependence) and side effects experienced (Table 3).

Table 5: Factors influencing the desire to stop vaping

Factor studied	P
Age of first use (over 25 years)	0,456
Frequency of vaping (consumption daily)	0,098
Feelings of anxiety secondary to vaping	0,472
Feeling addicted to e-cigarettes	0,98
Presence of side effects (somatic and psychological)	0,82
Beliefs about the use of electronic cigarettes (withdrawal, substitution)	0,002

DISCUSSION

Smoking is one of the greatest threats to public health. It is responsible for more than 8 million deaths a year. Tobacco control is a global health priority. (2) A number of medicinal and non-medicinal methods are used in this fight. The electronic cigarette, developed in the 2000s, is presented as an alternative to the traditional cigarette. However, its role in smoking cessation remains controversial, especially as its safety is debated. The aim of our work was to study the practices of e-cigarette users among medical students, to analyse their beliefs, experiences and expectations of this electronic device and to assess its influence on their smoking habits.

The strengths of our work

- Our study deals with a recent and rapidly evolving subject. It aims to understand the behaviour of vapers in order to pinpoint a phenomenon that is growing exponentially.

-       The population studied is made up of medical students, future key players in the fight against smoking.

The limits of our study

- The small size of the study population

- The responses were obtained using a self-questionnaire distributed via social networks, which means that the accuracy of the data cannot be guaranteed.

- This is a cross-sectional study, which does not allow us to follow students individually to see how they might change from vaping to smoking.

E-cigarette use is widespread throughout the world and the market is growing rapidly (3). According to a recent study published in 2022, the number of e-cigarette users has risen from 7 million in 2011 to 55 million in 2022, or 5.5% of adults (4). The ETINCEL-OFDT survey, a telephone survey on electronic cigarettes conducted in France in 2013 among a representative sample of 2,052 people. aged between 15 and 75, showed that 18% of French people have tried electronic cigarettes (i.e. between 8 and 9 million individuals) (5). There are no epidemiological data on the use of electronic cigarettes in Tunisia. Vape use often concerns a young population. French and international data show an explosion in the use of electronic cigarettes among teenagers(6). At university level, the study by Zarobkiewicz et al. estimates that 31.46% of students have already used e-cigarettes (37.28% (n=195) among non-medical university students and 25.87% (n=141) among medical university students) (7). According to La

Torre's multicentre study, the overall prevalence of smoking among medical students was estimated to be 29.3% higher than in the general population (8). The average age at which e-cigarette use began among French students was 20.8 years, according to Tavolacci (9). According to the results of our study, almost half the participants started vaping before the age of 25, with an average age of 26.25. Vaping is more common among men than women (5). According to a recent meta-analysis published in 2022, the prevalence of e-cigarette use was 12% among men and 8% among women. The same is true of our study. In fact, more than two-thirds of the participants were men. This could be explained by the higher prevalence of male smoking compared with female smoking throughout the world, but also in Tunisia, which suggests that men are more attracted than women to the world of tobacco, including the electronic cigarette (3,10), but this gap is tending to narrow, particularly in high-income countries where the prevalence of female smoking is increasing (11). According to the literature, there are several reasons for vaping, depending on the individual's smoking status. Most smokers start vaping with a view to giving up smoking (12,13). Their aim is often to stop smoking altogether, but they also use electronic cigarettes. To a lesser extent, vaping is motivated by the desire to stop smoking. reduction in tobacco consumption, but without complete cessation (5). For smokers, the availability of e-cigarettes over the counter and the fact that they do not require specialist medical supervision are the two main advantages of this device compared with nicotine substitutes. In addition, the use of this small device allows smokers to maintain their behavioural dependence (the routine gestures of smoking) and their physical dependence by meeting their daily nicotine requirements, thus avoiding the symptoms of withdrawal syndrome (5). It also produces a "throat hit" that smokers appreciate. This is the tingling sensation in the throat experienced when inhaling a product containing nicotine(14). Several studies have demonstrated the effectiveness of electronic cigarettes in helping the general population to reduce or stop smoking (15,16). However, given the paucity of information on its safety and efficacy, the public health authorities in France do not recommend it as a first-line smoking cessation aid (17). The French National Authority for Health (HAS) does not recommend it as a means of smoking cessation, although it does admit that, because it is much less toxic than a traditional cigarette, its use by smokers who have started vaping and want to stop smoking should not be discouraged, but they should consult their GP (18). The French Society of Respirology considers that the electronic cigarette is probably an effective aid in quitting smoking, provided that it is used only temporarily(19). Internationally, the WHO recommends that electronic cigarettes should not be used until their safety has been scientifically proven. Only a few countries, such as Brazil, Argentina and Singapore, have banned this product altogether; in other countries, such as Switzerland and Canada, only nicotine-free electronic cigarettes may be marketed (5). In our study, almost half the participants were smokers when they started vaping. Three quarters of them started using e-cigarettes to stop smoking. A minority achieved complete cessation. The other reasons for vaping found among smokers were the desire to save money, as vaping is even cheaper than smoking, or to avoid the inconveniences associated with smoking (bad breath, bad taste), or to reduce health risks without giving up smoking (5). Curiosity and the influence of peers are other reasons for vaping, particularly among non-smokers (18).

Several flavours are used in electronic cigarettes. According to the data in the literature, the most popular are fruit flavours, followed by sweet flavours (sweets, desserts) and mint- or menthol-based flavours (4). According to the study by Stenger et al, fruit flavour was the most commonly used (77.7%), followed by mint (9.1%) and tobacco flavour (5.5%) (6), which is consistent with the results of our study.

Fruit flavour was the most commonly used flavour in 58.1% of cases, followed by mint in 16.1%. The safety of electronic cigarettes is the subject of debate. The long-term consequences of vaping are not yet known, and it is the acute side effects that are best described. In most cases, these are benign symptoms such as throat irritation or a dry cough, or a slight increase in diastolic blood pressure that is much lower than that induced by conventional cigarettes. In addition, blood levels of carboxyhaemoglobin before and after using electronic cigarettes remain unchanged (18). Other more serious effects have been reported in the literature. These include an increased risk of infection. Vaping reduces the innate immune defences of the lungs by altering the antibacterial and viral functions of neutrophils and macrophages and reducing the protective function of mucus and the respiratory epithelium. It has also been shown that e-cigarette consumption can be responsible for a pneumopathy known as "vaping-related pneumopathy", defined by the presence of bilateral ground-glass pulmonary infiltrates, with or without alveolar condensation, occurring in a patient who has inhaled e-cigarette vapour within a few hours of smoking. 90 days, after ruling out respiratory infection and other plausible differential diagnoses depending on the medical context. This newly described entity is of variable severity, with mortality reported in between 2% and 6% of cases (4). However, the toxicity of electronic cigarettes is much lower than that of conventional cigarettes. It contains no tobacco and there is no combustion, so it releases no carbon monoxide, no significant quantities of fine solid particles (pro-inflammatory) or carcinogenic substances, unlike tobacco smoke (20). In the study by Moussa et al, the frequency of adverse effects was 28%, with coughing at the top of the list, followed by sore throat (12). Zarobkeiwicz states that 26.9% of e-cigarette users reported adverse effects such as headache, dryness of the mucous membranes, dyspnoea, coughing, sore throat and dizziness (7). In our study, mild adverse reactions were reported in 38.7% of cases, dominated by coughing, which is similar to the data in the literature.Scientists are also concerned about electronic cigarettes. They fear it could be a gateway to nicotine addiction and smoking. E-cigarettes contain an e-liquid made up of propylene glycol and vegetable glycerine, to which flavourings and nicotine are added in varying concentrations. Nicotine is known for its addictive effect. A non-smoker who uses an electronic nicotine inhaler may become addicted to nicotine and find it difficult to stop using it or become dependent on traditional tobacco products (18,21,22). In the study by STENGER et al, which looked at smoking in schools, 49.4% of the

3,319 students included had experimented with tobacco and electronic cigarettes, 11.6% of whom had vaped before smoking (6). In our study, almost half of the participants were not smokers of normal tobacco when they first experimented with electronic cigarettes, 15% of them wanted to switch to normal tobacco after starting to vapotage and 20% actually switched to smoked tobacco. To assess dependence on nicotine-delivering electronic cigarettes, some studies have used the Fagerström test. This is a six-question self-questionnaire with a total score ranging from 0 to 10. A score between 0 and 2 indicates no dependence, between 3 and 4 low dependence, between 5 and 6 medium dependence and above 10 high dependence (23). In an American study including 117 vapers, dependence was judged to be moderate in 45.5% of cases and was greater with vaping than with tobacco (24). In another Tunisian study, dependence on vaping was judged to be low in 35% of cases, moderate in 25% and high in 7.8% of cases, but less than dependence on tobacco (12). These results were qualified by other researchers. For example, Farsalinos et al have shown that with nicotine concentrations in e-liquids limited by law to 20 mg/ml, it is not possible to saturate nicotine receptors and create dependence (25). These figures should be treated with caution, however, as it has been shown that new electronic cigarette models can produce plasma nicotine levels approaching those produced by traditional cigarettes (18). The illegal market in e-cigarettes is also a cause for concern, as the nicotine concentrations in e-liquids are not controlled. In our study, 67.7% of participants used e-cigarettes on a daily basis, half of them increased the frequency of vaping over time and almost a third (35.5%) stopped using e-cigarettes but resumed at a later date. Half of the participants (45.2%) felt addicted to e-cigarettes. All these data point to a possible addictive effect of e-cigarettes.

Smoking is a real public health problem, with serious health consequences. Its prevalence in the general population remains high. Several medicinal and non-medicinal methods are available to combat smoking. The electronic cigarette (e-cigarette) is a new product whose use is increasing exponentially. Its role in smoking cessation is debated, and its safety remains a subject of controversy.In this context, we carried out a descriptive cross-sectional study using a self-administered questionnaire developed on Google Forms and distributed on social networks (Facebook). The aim was to study the practices and experiences of e-cigarette users among medical students, to analyse their expectations of this electronic device and to assess its influence on their smoking habits. Thirty-one students were included in our study with a mean age of 28±4 years, including 23 men and 8 women. The average age of first use of electronic cigarettes was 26.25±4.9 years. Sixteen participants were smoking regular tobacco when they started vaping. Twenty-one participants (67.7%) used e-cigarettes on a daily basis.Twenty participants (64.5%) intend to stop using electronic cigarettes. A further eleven (35.5%) have stopped using e-cigarettes but resumed at a later date.The concentration of nicotine in the e-liquid was 6 mg in 48.4% of cases. Almost a third of participants (38.7%) said they did not know the nicotine concentration in their e-cigarette. Fruit flavour was the flavour most used by study participants (58.1%), followed by mint flavour for 16.1% of subjects. Three participants used tobacco flavour. The reason for vaping among smokers was smoking cessation (12 participants),to find a better taste than tobacco (4 participants). The other reasons were curiosity (11 participants, 35.4%) and peer influence (4 participants, 12.9%). Nine smokers managed to reduce their tobacco consumption after using the e-cigarette and 3 participants managed to stop smoking completely.Three non-smokers wanted to switch to normal tobacco after starting to vapourise and 4 actually did switch to smoked tobacco. Mild adverse events, dominated by dry cough, were reported in 12 participants (38.7%).Around two-thirds of subjects (64.5%) thought that the electronic cigarette is a substitute for normal tobacco, and almost a third thought that the e-cigarette is more of a smoking cessation aid. Belief in the use of e-cigarettes was identified as a factor influencing the desire to stop vaping (p=0.002) and gender was correlated with the switch from using e-cigarettes to smoking tobacco (p=0.026). In the light of these results, the following conclusions and prospects emerge:

- Medical students, who will be major players in the fight against tobacco, need to be given more tobacco training. This training should be integrated into the clerkship studies and consolidated by seminars during the internship and residency. It should include information on the role of the electronic cigarette in the fight against smoking, emphasising that it cannot be prescribed by a doctor and that its use should only be considered on a temporary basis as part of the anti-smoking approach.

- Larger-scale studies are needed to analyse vape use among young people in general, in order to detect any misuse.

- Raising awareness among health authorities of the need for a legislative framework for the sale and use of e-cigarettes.

REFERENCES

1.Doll R, Peto R, Boreham J, Sutherland I. Mortality in relation to smoking: 50 years' observations on male British doctors. BMJ. 26 June 2004;328(7455):1519.

2.9789240077508-fre.pdf [Internet]. [cited 20 March 2024]. Available from: https://iris.who.int/bitstream/handle/10665/372570/9789240077508-fre.pdf?sequence=1

3.Tehrani H, Rajabi A, Ghelichi-Ghojogh M, Nejatian M, Jafari A. The prevalence of electronic cigarettes vaping globally: a systematic review and meta-analysis. Arch Public Health Arch Belg Sante Publique. 21 Nov 2022;80(1):240.

4.Georges M. Electronic cigarettes: news in 2022. Rev Mal Respir Actual. 1 Dec 2022;14(2, Supplement 2):2S418- 22.

5.Lermenier A, Palle C. Results of the ETINCEL-OFDT survey on electronic cigarettes [Internet]. 2014 [cited 25 Jul 2016]. Available from: http://www.ofdt.fr/BDD/publications/docs/eisxalu2.pdf

6.Stenger N, Chailleux E. Survey of e-cigarette and tobacco use in schools. Rev Mal Respir. Jan 2016;33(1):56- 62.

7.Zarobkiewicz MK, Wawryk-Gawda E, Woźniakowski MM, Sławiński MA, Jodłowska-Jędrych

B. Tobacco smokers and electronic cigarette users among Polish university students. Rocz Panstw Zakl Hig. 2016;67(1):75- 80.

8.La Torre G, Kirch W, Bes-Rastrollo M, Ramos RM, Czaplicki M, Gualano MR, et al. Tobacco use among medical students in Europe: results of a multicentre study using the Global Health Professions Student Survey. Public Health. Feb 2012;126(2):159- 64.

9.Tavolacci MP, Vasiliu A, Romo L, Kotbagi G, Kern L, Ladner J. Patterns of electronic cigarette use in current and ever users among college students in France: a cross-sectional study. BMJ Open. 27 May 2016;6(5):e011344.

10. Fakhfakh R, Hsairi M, Maalej M, Achour N. Smoking in Tunisia: behaviour and knowledge. 2002;

11. Clair C, Cornuz J, de Kleijn MJJ, Jaunin-Stalder N. Gender and disparities: the example of smoking. Rev Med Suisse. 10 June 2015;478:1298- 303.

12. E-cigarette dependence in former smoker: A Tunisian survey.

Chirine Moussa, Nour Mahmoud, Houda Rouis, Amel Khattab , Ines Zendah, Sonia Maâlej. Tunis Médicale [Internet]. 14 Oct 2023 [cited 17 Mar 2024];101(6). Available from: https://latunisiemedicale.com/index.php/tunismed/article/view/4275

13. Hummel K, Hoving C, Nagelhout GE, de Vries H, van den Putte B, Candel MJJM, et al. Prevalence and reasons for use of electronic cigarettes among smokers: Findings from the International Tobacco Control (ITC) Netherlands Survey. Int J Drug Policy. June 2015;26(6):601- 8.

14. Dubois G, Goullé JP, Costentin J, Allilaire JF, Dirheimer G, Dreux C, et al. Does the electronic cigarette allow society to get away from tobacco? Bull Académie Natl Médecine. 1 Feb 2015;199(2):363- 9.

15. Caponnetto P, Campagna D, Cibella F, Morjaria JB, Caruso M, Russo C, et al. EffiCiency and Safety of an eLectronic cigAreTte (ECLAT) as tobacco cigarettes substitute: a prospective 12-month randomized control design study. PloS One. 2013;8(6):e66317.

16. Bullen C, Howe C, Laugesen M, McRobbie H, Parag V, Williman J, et al. Electronic cigarettes for smoking cessation: a randomised controlled trial. Lancet Lond Engl. 16 Nov 2013;382(9905):1629- 37.

17. Moyou-Mogo R. The role of vaping in smoking cessation. JMV-J Médecine Vasc. 1 March 2023;48:S40- 1.

18. Charton P. The role of electronic cigarettes in smoking cessation.

19. Vape-SFT_SPLF-MoissansTabac-20191101-ok.pdf [Internet]. [cited 17 March 2024]. Available from: https://splf.fr/wp-content/uploads/2019/11/Vape-SFT_SPLF- MoissansTabac-20191101-ok.pdf

20. Sci-Hub | The electronic cigarette: a new tool in the approach to smokers? Archives Des Maladies Du Coeur et Des Vaisseaux - Pratique, 2014(229), 39-42 | 10.1016/s1261- 694x(14)70651-0 [Internet]. [cited 18 March 2024]. Available from: https://sci-hub.st/10.1016/s1261-694x(14)70651-0

21. Grana RA. Electronic cigarettes: a new nicotine gateway? J Adolesc Health Off Publ Soc Adolesc Med. Feb 2013;52(2):135- 6.

22. Dautzenberg B, Birkui P, Noël M, Dorsett J, Osman M, Dautzenberg MD. E-Cigarette: A New Tobacco Product for Schoolchildren in Paris. Open J Respir Dis. 22 Feb 2013;3(1):21- 4.

23. Underner M, Le Houezec J, Perriot J, Peiffer G. Les tests d'évaluation de la dépendance tabagique. Rev Mal Respir. Apr

2012;29(4):462- 74.

24. Johnson JM, Muilenburg JL, Rathbun SL, Yu X, Naeher LP, Wang JS. Elevated Nicotine Dependence Scores among Electronic Cigarette Users at an Electronic Cigarette Convention. J Community Health. Feb 2018;43(1):164- 74.

25. Farsalinos KE, Spyrou A, Tsimopoulou K, Stefopoulos C, Romagna G, Voudris V. Nicotine absorption from electronic cigarette use: comparison between first and new-generation devices. Sci Rep. 26 Feb 2014;4:4133.

ELECTRONIC CIGARETTE USE AMONG MEDICAL

STUDENTS

SUMMARY

Introduction :

Smoking is one of the leading causes of preventable disease and premature death in the world. Tobacco control and prevention are priorities in the fight against this scourge. Electronic cigarettes are seen by the general public as a way of helping people to stop smoking. However, this remains a controversial issue.

Methods :

Cross-sectional descriptive study of medical students in Tunisia. The aim of this study is to investigate the practices and experiences of e-cigarette users among medical students, to analyse their expectations of this electronic device and to assess its influence on their smoking habits.

Results :

Our population comprised 31 subjects with a mean age of 28±4 years and a sex ratio of 2.87. Smoking tobacco was present in 74.2% of cases. Consumption of other psychoactive substances was noted in 16.1% of cases (5 participants).Fifteen participants (48.3%) had experimented with electronic cigarettes before the age of 25. Fifteen participants (48.3%) were not regular tobacco smokers when they started vaping. Twenty-one participants (37.7%) used e-cigarettes on a daily basis, with 64.5% using them several times a day. Almost half of the participants (51.6%, n=16) increased the frequency of vaping over time. At the time of initiation of vaping, sixteen participants were normal cigarette smokers (51.6%), twelve participants (39%) started vaping with a view to giving up smoking. Nine of them succeeded in reducing their tobacco consumption after using the e-cigarette and 3 participants succeeded in giving up smoking completely. Fifteen people were not smokers of normal tobacco when they first tried the electronic cigarette, and four of them actually switched to smoked tobacco. Around two-thirds of subjects (64.5%) thought that the electronic cigarette is a substitute for normal tobacco, and almost a third thought that the e-cigarette is more of a smoking cessation aid.

The analytical study concluded that the number of cigarettes consumed per day was correlated with daily vape use (p=0.044) and that gender was a factor associated with switching from e-cigarettes to smoked tobacco (p=0.026). Belief in the use of e-cigarettes was also found to be a factor influencing the desire to stop vaping (p=0.002).

Conclusion:

Smoking is responsible for over 8 million deaths a year. The fight against smoking is vital. Medical students, who will play a key role in the fight against smoking, need to be given more training in tobaccology.

Key word : Smoking, E-cigarette, Medical students, Smoking cessation

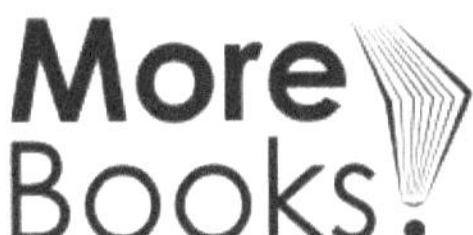
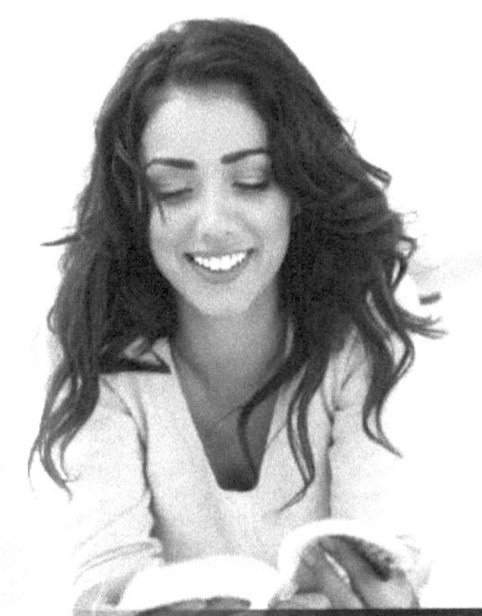

I want morebooks!

Buy your books fast and straightforward online - at one of world's fastest growing online book stores! Environmentally sound due to Print-on-Demand technologies.

Buy your books online at
www.morebooks.shop

Kaufen Sie Ihre Bücher schnell und unkompliziert online – auf einer der am schnellsten wachsenden Buchhandelsplattformen weltweit! Dank Print-On-Demand umwelt- und ressourcenschonend produziert.

Bücher schneller online kaufen
www.morebooks.shop

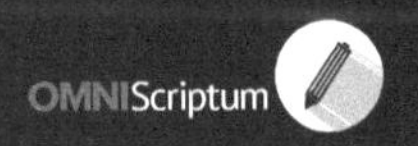

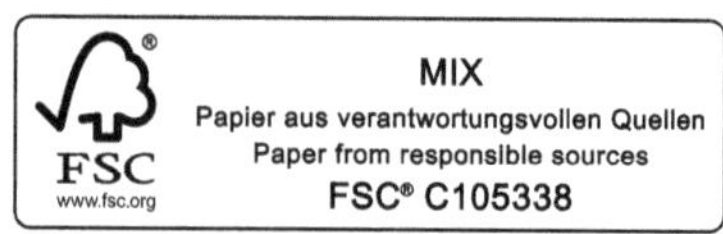

Printed by Books on Demand GmbH, Norderstedt / Germany